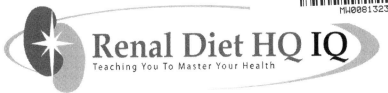

ALTERNATIVE TREATMENT OPTIONS FOR CHRONIC KIDNEY FAILURE

Book 12

By Mathea Ford, RD/LD

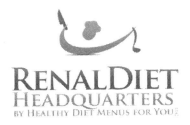

PURPOSE AND INTRODUCTION

What I have found through the emails and requests of my readers is that it is difficult to find information about a pre-dialysis kidney lifestyle that is actionable. I want you to know that is what I intend to provide in all my books.

I wrote this book with you in mind: the person with kidney problems who does not know where to start or can't seem to get the answers that you need from other sources. This book will provide information that is applicable to a predialysis kidney disease lifestyle.

Who am I? I am a registered dietitian in the USA who has been working with kidney patients for my entire 15 + years of experience. Find all my books on Amazon on my author page: http://www.amazon.com/Mathea-Ford/e/B008E1E7IS/

My goals are simple – to give some answers and to create an understanding of what is typical. In this series of 12 books, I will take you through the different parts of being a person with pre-dialysis kidney disease. It will not necessarily be what happens in your case, as everyone is an individual. I may simplify things in an effort to write them so that I feel you can learn the most from the information. This may mean that I don't say the exact things that your doctor would say. If you don't understand, please ask your doctor.

I want you to know, I am not a medical doctor and I am not aware of your particular condition. Information in this book is current as of publication, but may or may not have changed. This book is not meant to substitute for medical treatment for you, your friends, your caregivers, or your family members. You should not base treatment decisions solely on what is contained in this book. Develop your treatment plan with your doctors, nurses and the other medical professionals on your team. I recommend that you double-check any information with your medical team to verify if it applies to you. In other words, I am not responsible for your medical care. I am providing this book for information and entertainment purposes, not medical diagnoses. Please consult with your doctor about any questions that you have about your particular case. © 2014 Renal Diet Headquarters, www.renaldiethq.com , All Rights Reserved. No reproduction without author's written permission

TABLE OF CONTENTS

INTRODUCTION

Traditional treatment of chronic kidney disease usually includes dietary and lifestyle changes, but in some cases includes dialysis. For some individuals, a transplant is an option. However, both treatments are serious medical procedures. Recovery from a kidney transplant can be long and challenging, since it *is* major surgery. Sometimes it can be hard to find the right donor, and the dialysis and transplant waiting process can be difficult. Dialysis, while unquestionably valuable, can be a lengthy procedure that's expensive and time consuming. It's something that most people aim to avoid when they are able to.

Some individuals with chronic kidney disease are able to find alternative treatments that are helpful both in treating the symptoms of the disease and even in preventing it from worsening. Many of these alternative treatments help them postpone surgery, or even avoid it altogether. Additional benefits of alternative treatments for kidney disease include:

- Stress Management

- Inflammation reduction

- Stabilizing creatinine levels

- A decrease in swelling (edema)

- Lowering blood pressure

- Pain management – Reduction in severity and frequency

- Flushing out toxins from kidneys

Some of the alternative therapies individuals have found helpful in terms of kidney disease include lifestyle changes, herbs and supplements, dietary measures, stress relieving activities, CranioSacral therapy, and Traditional Chinese medicine (TCM). The treatments work by allowing the kidneys to rest and reducing the amount of work they have to do and by activating other "cleansing" organs, such as the liver and skin, in order to help support the kidneys.

In some cases, the alternative treatments are complementary to the medications and treatments that the patient are already receiving, ensuring that the patient is getting the utmost relief possible. Many of the therapies can be used in conjunction with one another. In other cases, the patient might chose to use an alternative treatment in replacement of a more traditional approach. In the following book, we'll talk about some of the alternative treatments for chronic kidney disease and how the treatments are done. Of course, before starting on any alternative treatment, please talk to your doctor first. Never stop taking a medication or start taking any supplement before speaking to your physician.

INFLAMMATION AND CHRONIC ILLNESS

One of the reasons that alternative medications work is because of their ability to treat the inflammation in the body. They help to reduce the stress response and irritation in our body and allow it to work better.

Inflammation is the body's reaction to some harmful effect in the body, and it is important to the healing process. Our body has certain cells that react when our body has damage. These cells are the body's attempt to protect ourselves and remove harmful cells, irritants, and pathogens that enter our body or are created in our body. This is the beginning of the healing process for our cells and our bodies, to rid the cells of the damage and protect us through inflammation.

Acute inflammation starts quickly in an area – like a cut or scrape – and quickly can become severe. But other types of inflammation happen in our bodies, and when they continue to be irritated over time it is called chronic inflammation. The build-up of plaque in our arteries from cholesterol is partly from irritation and inflammation which then heals over the imbedded fatty tissues and blocks the artery. To be sure, our bodies need to do this process or we would not heal and having an open wound would be bad. But when it happens for long periods of time, it is bad. Inflammation needs to be regulated in our bodies. Reducing inflammation if it's chronic can be helpful, but you need to allow the healing process to happen as well.

So, in your kidneys, it's small amounts of damage over time that lead to reducing the ability of your nephrons to function. This is an inflammatory process that your body has going on all the time. And many of these alternative therapies are focused on trying to help your body reduce the inflammation caused by the chronic problems. So they reduce swelling or relax you and that can help with dealing with inflammation. That's not all they do, they can affect you other ways, but it's important to understand that a large part of the healing comes from controlling the inflammation.

FINDING TREATMENT OUTSIDE OF STANDARD MEDICINE

Although it's important to follow any instructions your doctor gives you and to make sure you report any changes to your medical team, it's still possible to find treatment complementary to your medical team. When you are seeking treatment, it's important to understand what your individual goals are. Are you seeking pain relief? Symptomatic relief? Are you looking for ways to eliminate stress? Are you trying to avoid surgery or postpone going on dialysis? The clearer you are in your own health goals, the more your own doctor will be able to work with you and the more informed you'll be when you're researching the additional different treatment alternatives that exist.

The treatments can be complementary and don't have to contradict one another. A variety of health professionals are able to offer alternative treatments for kidney disease and many of these are professionally trained and educated. Naturopaths and chiropractors, for instance, are often sought for relief and treatment; both of these fields require extensive knowledge of their particular subject matter, and sometimes accept insurance.

Naturopaths can help you take a holistic approach to your health when it comes to controlling kidney disease and its symptoms and preventing the disease from worsening. Naturopaths are trained to look at herbs, diet, and lifestyle changes. They combine the understanding of nature with the accuracy of contemporary science. Naturopathic medicine focuses on holistic health, meaning that it looks at the body as a whole and doesn't just focus on the disease at hand- in this case kidney disease. It offers a comprehensive diagnosis and treatment, and many individuals feel it is superior to modern medicine which tends to focus on the ailment and not the whole person.

Naturopathic physicians aid the body in being able to restore its health and proper workings by creating an overall healing environment, inside and out. When a naturopathic physician treats a patient, they take their genetics, mental health, environment, and physical health into consideration. They might also encourage the individual to focus on their spiritual health, since part of the holistic approach includes spirituality.

So where does one go to find a naturopath? You can find naturopathic physicians in a range of places, including hospitals, clinics, and their own private practices. Despite the fact that these are considered, in many circles, to be "alternative healthcare providers," they are still highly educated. To be considered a qualified naturopathic physician, the individual must undergo painstaking training and education. A good physician, even in naturopathy, will be licensed and will continue to have ongoing training throughout his or her career.

Naturopathic physicians are trained to work with prescription drugs, but they don't use them unless it's absolutely necessary. Instead, they try to rely on natural medicine for their healing. You may or may not be prescribed any prescription medication if you go to a naturopath. Some of their diagnostic and therapeutic modalities include: laboratory diagnostic testing, botanical medicine, naturopathic manipulative therapy, nutritional medicine, counseling, homeopathy, acupuncture, IV therapy, and natural childbirth. They can do minor surgery but are not considered surgeons. For instance, they might stitch up a wound but you wouldn't go to them for knee surgery. Some of the ailments they are known for treating include adrenal fatigue, chronic fatigue syndrome, hormonal imbalances, and chronic pain. They can also be helpful in treating kidney disease and some of its symptoms.

Herbal healers, or herbalists, can create solutions that might help flush out the kidneys and control symptoms associated with kidney disease. Herbalism has been practiced for thousands of years and remains popular today. Herbalism is often associated with traditional Chinese medicine, although your herbalist may not be linked to the Asian arts.

Treating certain ailments with natural herbs is a part of naturopathy, although not all herbalists are naturopaths. Although an herbal healer doesn't have to be licensed, some are. An herbalist can pursue a career in the field either formally or informally. Some herbalists, for instance, are folk herbalists and work within a small group of people, such as an organization. Professional herbalists, however, have recognized credentials that may have come from a university. Certification can come from a peer-reviewed organization such as the Natural Healing College, The American Herbalists Guild, or the National Institute of Medical Herbalists. Other herbalists practice as naturopathic physicians and fulfill clinical and academic requirements.

A chiropractor is another medical professional that is often used for alternative treatments. They use what is termed as a "spinal manipulation" or "chiropractic adjustment" to help treat and prevent a multitude of health problems, from back pain to chronic sinus issues. By manually applying force to the joints and nerves that are restricted, the adjustment is meant to re-establish joint mobility. Oftentimes, the joints become restricted due to an injury to the surrounding tissue. This can be caused by repetitive stress, such as poor posture, or lifting something heavy.

In terms of kidney disease, alignments have been known to help reduce swelling, flush out toxins, and increase energy. For those who experience lower back pain associated with kidney disease, going to the chiropractor might be beneficial as well. Chiropractors believe the body's systems work in relation to one another other. As a result, kidney disease could be affected by interference to the nervous system. Using chiropractic adjustments in addition to other holistic procedures might offer symptomatic relief and help stop the disease from getting worse.

Chiropractors must undergo training and be licensed in order to practice. They use clinical examination, X-rays, laboratory testing, and additional diagnostic interventions to assess their patients and figure out which treatments will suit them best and how often those treatments are needed. If necessary, a chiropractor can refer a patient to additional health care providers if they feel progress is not being made in your care.

Some of these healthcare providers might be covered in the cost of your healthcare insurance while others might not be. Chiropractors can be covered under some plans, although you might need a referral from your primary care physician and you may be limited by the number of visits your insurance will pay for. Other alternative treatments are generally not covered but it never hurts to call and ask your healthcare plan first.

Of course, if you are having any new symptoms it's always important not to try to self-diagnose. Always tell your doctor, even if you feel like the concern may be unfounded. Whether the symptom came on suddenly or has developed over time, it's better to err on the side of caution.

DIETARY CHANGES

In terms of alternative medicine and diet, before embarking upon any dietary changes, always talk to your dietitian or healthcare provider before adding any new foods to your diet or eliminating anything that was part of your kidney diet plan.

There's no doubt that the diet plays a big part in our overall health and you can't deny the fact that the food we consume is integral to the way our body performs and functions. By making simple dietary changes some patients have been able to find relief from symptoms associated with kidney disease and even delay the need for dialysis.

Some food choices can be added to a diet in order to help flush out the kidneys, slowing down the progression of kidney disease, preventing kidney stones, and reducing the swelling that is often a symptom of kidney disease. Some of these food products include: apple cider vinegar, cucumber juice, and cornsilk. In addition, increasing your water intake so that it's at least 8-12 glasses per day can be helpful in flushing out the toxins through the urine. (Although in advanced renal failure it's often advised to decrease your water intake so you should follow any instructions that your doctor advises in terms of water intake.) There are also foods that should be avoided for those with kidney disease. These include foods that are rich in protein, salt and potassium. For some patients, sticking to a kidney disease diet is often suggested by their doctor or dietitian. An appropriate diet can help control the progress of the disease and also have other benefits.

SUPER FOODS FOR YOUR KIDNEYS

Eating a balanced diet is important. There are also super foods, that can be helpful in promoting good kidney health and are used in alternative treatments for kidney disease. These "super foods" mostly have to do with oxidation and free radicals. Oxidation produces energy and is a normal chemical process.

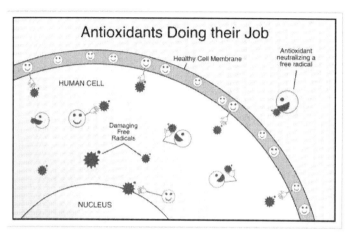

Sometimes, though, it can cause free radicals and these are unbalanced molecules that can roam freely around the body and damage tissue, cells, and proteins. Free radicals can cause damage that can lead to everything from premature signs of aging to cancer. Super foods, however, contain antioxidants and these can help neutralize the free radicals and slow the rate of oxidation that is caused by them.

Some of the most common antioxidants found in super foods include lycopene, flavonoids, and vitamins C, and E.

To make the concept of antioxidants and free radicals more clear, think about free radicals like the ghosts in the Pac-Man® game, running around your body. And antioxidants are like Pac-Man® himself, munching them down.

The following super foods have been found beneficial for those suffering from kidney disease due to their antioxidant properties or for other properties as described below:

Apple Cider Vinegar: Apple cider vinegar (often abbreviated as ACV) is probably one of the most popular folk remedies out there and is used to treat everything from sinus infections to constipation. It can also be effective in the breaking down of kidney stones. The acid in ACV works by disintegrating the calculi that's formed by calcium in the kidneys. ACV also has a diuretic effect and this can be helpful in flushing the kidneys out. The ACV's antibacterial properties help prevent and heal bacterial infections. Apple cider vinegar is a lot more palatable than drinking straight vinegar. Some people are able to drink it alone, without adding anything to it. When doing this, you don't want to drink anymore than 1-2 tablespoons at a time, but try to do it at least once a day. You can also dilute the ACV in water, hot or cold.

A quick and easy recipe for making some Apple Cider Vinegar Limeade –

1. Take a 1 quart jar and add the following:

    a. 2 Tbsp Apple Cider Vinegar

    b. 1 Tbsp Lime Juice Concentrate

    c. 4 tsp Truvia or other sweetener (or to taste)

2. Fill with ice and water for remaining part of jar. Cover with lid, shake, and drink. You can keep the beverage in the refrigerator for the day and drink throughout.

Cornsilk: The corn cob tassels, which are usually thrown away, might actually be valuable in treating kidney and urinary infections. In addition, they could help prevent the formation of kidney stones and even help eliminate swelling caused by kidney disease. Cornsilk can be used to ease certain types of pain found within the urinary tract, too, and is frequently used to treat pain from kidney stones. The best way to eat cornsilk is to make a sweet tea out of it by boiling it in water for several minutes.

Cucumbers: Cucumbers have a high water content which makes them ideal for kidney disease patients. It has also been discovered that drinking cucumber and carrot juice is a powerful natural home remedy for individuals facing kidney failure. When patients are suffering from a declining ability for kidneys to filter, dangerous toxins and waste can build up in the kidneys and bloodstream. This can lead to many different health issues, including anemia and vomiting. Cucumbers are a natural cleanser and can help the kidneys flush out the wastes, toxins, and acids more efficiently. In addition, a lot of patients suffer from kidney and bladder stones. Although these can be benign, they are still incredibly painful and irritating. Cucumbers can be helpful in dissolving these stones and, with their diuretic properties, help flush them out through the urine. The cucumbers can be eaten raw or with some apple cider vinegar.

Red bell peppers: Red bell peppers are good for kidney health since they're low in potassium. They also contain a lot of vitamins A, C, and B6, as well as folic acid and fiber. In addition, they provide the body with lycopene, an antioxidant, which can protect against some kinds of cancer. Red bell peppers are easy to add to the diet since they can be added to lots of different types of dishes, from raw salads to grilled vegetable plates. They don't lose any of their potency if they're cooked.

Red Grapes: Flavanoids, which help prevent oxidation and blood clots as well as being heart-healthy, cause the deep color in red grapes. Reservatrol, one of the flavanoids, might even boost the production of nitric oxide. Nitric oxide can encourage the muscle relaxation in blood vessels which can cause better blood flow. In addition, flavonoids can help prevent inflammation and this is important in kidney disease. To get the most flavanoids, go for the red grapes that have the deepest colors. Grapes make an excellent snack or can be tossed in a salad. They can also be added to a juicer to make a drink or frozen for a cool treat.

Strawberries: Strawberries make a very good sweet dessert and they're healthy, too. They have 2 kinds of phenols, anthocyanins and ellagitannins. The anthocyananins are potent antioxidants and give them their red color. They help protect the cell structures and the body from oxidative damage. Strawberries also contain vitamin C and manganese. They're known for their anti-inflammatory properties, too. Strawberries can be eaten alone for a healthy snack or tossed in salads. They can be made into purees, frozen, or squeezed into juice.

Pineapple: Pineapple is a sweet fruit that can make a nice dessert and it has a natural enzyme thanks to its bromelain. As a result, it is able to fight inflammation. As far as kidney disease is concerned, bromelain might be able to reduce any amyloid, a kind of protein deposit in the kidneys. Bromelain is most potent when it's taken along with the spice turmeric since turmeric has anti-inflammatory properties.

Cranberries: Both cranberries and cranberry juice have been used to treat urinary tract infections for a long time. Cranberries help with urinary tract infections since, by making the urine more acidic, it won't stay in the bladder for as long. Cranberries contain high levels of vitamin C as well. They also contain anthocyanins, a powerful anti-inflammatory compound. All of these properties are important for the kidneys to work properly and for the blood pressure to be properly balanced. According to a study published in the *British Journal of Urology* in 2003, cranberries, and specifically pure cranberry juice, can even prevent and dissolve kidney stones. When drinking cranberry juice you should drink pure juice and not diluted or cocktail juice. Cranberries can also be eaten raw or made into cranberry sauce or salad.

Cauliflower: Cauliflower is a cruciferous vegetable that's high in vitamin C and a good source of folate and fiber. Half a cup only contains 9 mg of sodium yet has a lot of indoles, glucosinolates and thiocyanates which are compounds that help the liver neutralize toxic substances that could cause harm to cell membranes and DNA. Cauliflower can be steamed or boiled and eaten alone or served raw as part of a raw vegetable tray. It can also be mashed and served as a low-fat substitute for mashed potatoes.

Olive oil: Olive oil contains many healthy properties which makes it a very good cooking choice. It has less than 1 mg of sodium per tablespoon and is a good source of oleic acid, an anti-inflammatory fatty acid. The monounsaturated fat found in olive oil helps protect against oxidation. Olive oil contains polyphenols and antioxidants that also help prevent inflammation and oxidation. Some research shows that those who use a lot of olive oil, such as Mediterranean cultures, have lower instances of certain forms of cancers and heart disease. It's best to use extra virgin (also called EVOO) or virgin olive oil since they have more antioxidants. Olive oil can be used in place of regular vegetable oil or used to drizzle over vegetables and bread.

Fish: You probably already know by now how healthy most types of fish are for you. In fact, the American Heart Association suggests that you eat fish at least twice a week. Fish offers the good kind of protein plus it has anti-inflammatory fats referred to as omega-3s. These help fight medical conditions like heart disease and cancer and can help lower LDL cholesterol, which is the bad kind, while raising the good kind (HDL). The fish that is highest in omega-3s are herring, salmon, rainbow trout, and albacore tuna.

Onions: Onions belong to the Allium family. They're often used to flavor dishes, although they're also healthy food items in their own rights and they're useful to include in a kidney disease diet. Just ½ cup of onions contain only 3 mg of sodium yet are rich in flavanoids, nature's chemicals that help prevent fatty materials from depositing in the blood vessels. They also contain a potent antioxidant called quercetin. This helps prevent heart disease as well as protects against some forms of cancers. Onions don't have a lot of potassium, another fact that's good for those with kidney disease. Onions are healthy regardless of the color they come in. They can be eaten raw or cooked with other foods in order to add flavor to them.

Berries: Berries of all different kinds are healthy to eat, especially if they're bright in color. Raspberries and blueberries are especially important for those with kidney disease since they contain anthocyanins, the compound that provides them with their color.

Anthocyanins contain lots of nutrients that can reduce inflammation. These berries also contain a lot of vitamin C, manganese, phosphorus, and potassium. Raspberries contain ellagic acid, a compound which neutralizes free radicals.

Egg whites: Just two egg whites contain as much as 7 grams of protein, making them excellent substitutes for meat when you're trying to get enough protein for the day. They also contain a lot of essential amino acids. For those with kidney disease, they have the protein you need without a lot of phosphorus. You can eat fresh egg whites or the powdered kind. You can use the egg whites to make omelets, a sandwich, or an egg salad sandwich.

Apples: Apples are known to reduce bad cholesterol levels and protect against heart disease, proving that an apple a day really can help keep the doctor away. They can also help reduce the risk of certain types of cancer and help regulate the bowels and ease constipation. Apples are high in fiber and contain anti-inflammatory compounds. Apples can be eaten in a variety of ways. They may be eaten raw for a snack, baked, included in dessert dishes, juiced, or made into applesauce.

Cherries: Cherries might be small, but that doesn't mean they aren't powerful. When eaten on a daily basis, it's been shown that they have the ability to reduce inflammation. They also have antioxidant properties and can help protect the heart, thanks to their phytochemicals. Cherries can be eaten fresh and raw or cooked and eaten in dessert dishes such as cherry jubilee or cherry pie.

Cabbage: Cabbage is a cruciferous vegetable. It contains 60 mg of potassium and 9 mg of phosphorus per ½ cup. It also contains a lot of phytochemicals which help break up free radicals. Phytochemicals can also fight against cancer and encourage good heart health. Cabbage is a good source of vitamins C, K, and B6. It contains folic acid and does not contain a lot of potassium. Raw cabbage can be eaten in coleslaw. Cabbage can also be steamed or boiled. Some people also stuff cabbage with meat and bake it with other herbs and seasonings for a meal.

Garlic: Garlic is a little bit of a wonder food. It can be used to lower cholesterol, reduce inflammation, and even help fight infections. In a study reported in the *Iranian Journal of Kidney Diseases* in 2011, it was discovered that the juice from garlic could drastically prevent renal reperfusion-induced functional damages. When the kidneys have a short time with lack of oxygen due to damaged tissue, then the tissue recovers and receives blood and nutrients, it is possible to have some additional damage caused by the return of blood flow. This is called reperfusion injury.

Garlic has the ability to boost the immune system which might be able to reduce damage that has been done to the kidneys. It also has an antioxidant effect and this can eliminate the free radicals which could cause kidney disease in the first place. Since garlic is a diuretic, it's been known to relieve water and sodium retention which can help with edema, a common symptom associated with kidney disease. This can also put less pressure on the artery walls and even lower blood pressure. Several studies have shown that garlic is effective in protecting the kidneys from dangerous heavy metals such as lead and cadmium. Garlic can be used to flavor a range of dishes, from pastas to meat dishes. It can also be roasted and spread on different kinds of bread and be used as a replacement for salt.

ADDITIONAL FOODS
Additional foods that have been found beneficial for those with kidney disease include radishes, beets, and asparagus. Radishes are a natural kidney cleanser and can help the kidneys get rid of harmful substances; beets are excellent at treating high blood pressure and heart problems which can be common with those suffering from kidney disease; and asparagus is good for treating symptoms of diabetes- one of the leading causes of kidney problems and kidney failure.

It's important to discuss with your renal dietitian about incorporating any of these foods into a healthy eating plan. Although these are all healthy foods, they might not be for everyone, especially if you have a food allergy to one of them. In addition, there might be a rare case where a certain food might cause an interaction with a medication that you're already on so it's important to discuss any dietary changes with your doctor.

FOODS TO LIMIT:
It's possible to prevent or delay some health issues associated with chronic kidney disease by avoiding or limiting certain foods that are high in sodium, phosphorus, and potassium. In addition, consuming too much protein can overburden the kidneys as well. Foods that contain a lot of protein can break down into nitrogen and creatinine which are waste products that healthy kidneys are normally able to remove from the blood but that unhealthy kidneys have trouble removing. As a result, the waste can build up and cause additional health problems and more disease.

The following is a short list of foods you should try to limit if possible to reduce your symptoms.

Protein: If you already suffer from kidney disease but aren't on dialysis yet, then it's important to limit your intake of foods that are high in protein. These types of food produce uric acid and this is one of the toxins the kidneys must eliminate. When the body's protein level is too high, the kidneys must work harder to deplete the surplus uric acid. It's recommended to only eat about 6-8 ounces of protein per day with pre dialysis kidney disease. Some examples of food that are rich in protein include:

Chicken

Pork

Beef

Fish

Sodium: The amount of sodium you consume on a daily basis should be limited as well. Too much sodium can cause edema, or excess swelling. Sodium can also increase your blood pressure. Highly processed foods, and canned products, can contain high levels of sodium.

It's best to try to choose products that are labeled "low-sodium" or "sodium-free." Your goal should be to keep your complete sodium intake to around 1,500 milligrams or less per day. You can find the amount of sodium on the labels of the food items you buy. There are also alternative items for most popular foods. For instance, instead of salt try salt-free herb seasonings and rather than canned vegetables buy frozen vegetables.

- Don't add salt to your food during the time you cook or when you are eating.
- Cook with herbs, lemon juice or salt-free spices.
- Use fresh or frozen vegetables instead of canned.
- If using canned vegetables, drain and rinse them first.
- Try to avoid processed meats such as bacon and deli-style meats.
- Eat fresh fruits and vegetables instead of crackers.
- Make your own fresh soups instead of eating canned ones using low sodium broth.
- Avoid high-sodium condiments such as soy sauce, teriyaki, and ketchup.

Potassium: You can find potassium in a lot of vegetables and fruits, especially bananas and tomatoes. Although we need potassium in order to function properly, too much can cause further damage to your kidneys. Without proper amounts of potassium, your heart and muscles will grow weak. Your physician should be able to check your blood to see that your level is within its normal range. If it's too high, you might need to avoid some foods that are high in potassium. It's possible to reduce the amount of potassium in some vegetables, like potatoes, by soaking them for a few hours before you cook them.

If you do need to substitute some fruits and vegetables for those with lower potassium contents then consider switching out oranges for apples, kiwi for plums, bananas for strawberries, tomatoes for cabbage, and cauliflower for potatoes.

Phosphorus: Phosphorus is a mineral and too much of it can take calcium away from your bones. This can make them weak and literally cause them to break. Foods that are high in phosphorus include nuts, peas, cheese, peanut butter, milk, dried beans, and canned ice tea. Some individuals end up having to take a phosphate binder such as calcium carbonate to control the phosphorus in their blood. These help bind the phosphorus while it's in the stomach so it gets passed through the stool instead of going into the bloodstream. Low-phosphorus substitutes include: popcorn, green beans, sherbet, pasta, rice, rice cereal, root beer, and lemonade mixes.

Fats: Fats are not all bad, since they give the body energy and help regulate blood pressure and other heart functions. Some fats really are healthier than others, however. Trans-fats and saturated fats can raise blood cholesterol levels and clog blood vessels, and this is not good for anyone, especially the person with kidney disease. Saturated fats can be found in animal products such as whole milk, red meat, and butter-products that are solid when they're at room temperature. On the other hand, trans-fats are usually in commercial baked goods such as cakes and fried foods such as French fries. When choosing oils, try to pick vegetable oil like corn oil over animal fats (butter). Hydrogenated vegetable oils should be avoided since they have trans-fats so this means that monosaturated fats such as olive oil are ideal

A portion controlled meal plan is important for overall good health when managing kidney disease. When treating kidney disease, it might even help prevent further kidney damage which is why it's so important in alternative treatment plans. It's important to work with your dietitian and educate yourself in order to make a meal plan that's right for you and helps you get the minerals and nutrients that you need.

TRADITIONAL CHINESE MEDICINE

In the past, traditional Chinese medicine (TCM) has been used to treat a variety of medical conditions, from chronic pain to sinusitis and diabetes. It can also be used to help relieve the symptoms of chronic kidney disease. Some of symptoms that TCM might be able to alleviate include both high and low blood pressure, pain, insomnia, fatigue, weakness, and edema. There are different elements of TCM. These are medicated baths, herbs, acupoint dressing therapy, acupuncture, Micro-Chinese Medicine Osmotherapy. Micro-Chinese Medicine Osmotherapy is an external application which can help patients avoid any further deterioration and protect their remaining kidney functions.

Traditional Chinese medicine focuses on controlling the patient's blood pressure, which may be high. TCM believes that this might help prevent future kidney deterioration so controlling blood pressure important. In addition, it's important to protect the nephrons and toxic retention and to control the diet. In fact, controlling the diet is essential treatment with TCM. Patients will follow a diet that consists of low protein with adequate calories and low salt. Enemas are common to help purge viscera to help get rid of toxins.

Chinese herbal medicated baths help eliminate toxins and get rid of itching. These are good for individuals who have edema and those who are suffering from end-stage kidney failure. Herbs that are often used in the herbal medicated baths include: duckweed, herba periliae, cassi twig, and cortex dictamni.

The acupoint dressing therapy includes applying medicine on an acupoint and treating the kidney disease internally. The herbal medicines, which are chosen by an herbalist, are mixed with a penetrating agent and applied on the acupoint. This helps delay the deterioration of the renal function. Some of the common medications/herbs include monkshood slice, peach seed, safflower and Coptidis rhizome.

These treatments are all treatments that are carried out by a trained herbalists and not something that the patient puts together on their own. Of course, the patient will bathe themselves. A trained herbalist will understand which herbs work together best and which ones are best in the remedy of kidney disease. As previously mentioned, an herbalist generally has specialized training from a recognized naturopathy school.

MICRO-CHINESE MEDICINE OSMOTHERAPY TREATMENT

Micro-Chinese Medicine Osmotherapy is based on TCM with advanced medical technology. Depending on the patient's illness, sometimes medication will be prescribed. They will be ground down into fine powder and placed in small bags which are soaked into a solution and situated under the individual's back right renal areas. On the other side, the bags are connected with osmoscopes which help promote the absorption of active ingredients.

With this osmosis device, the herbal ingredients permeate through skin into damaged kidney tissues. The herbal ingredients help dilate blood vessels and enter into the bloodstreams. They then nourish the affected kidney tissues, helping to prevent future kidney damage.

ACUPUNCTURE

Acupuncture is very important when it comes to TCM. It's becoming increasingly popular in the western world and is used to treat a wide variety of diseases, from chronic pain to allergies.

Acupuncture involves placing tiny needles on the surface of the body according to the individual's illness. The places where the needles are located are called "acupoints" or sometimes "trigger points." They correspond with the body's internal organs and immune system. In acupuncture, it is believed that the acupoints help stimulate the body's natural healing abilities.

Acupuncture might help with kidney disease in a couple of different ways. In order for the kidneys to function properly, there must be good blood flow to all of the organs. If there is a deficiency of blood in one or both of the kidneys, then renal ischemia can occur. Renal ischemia is damage from a lack of oxygen to tissues. Likewise, another common concern in CKD is when the tissues in the body don't have enough oxygen, usually caused by insufficient oxygen in the blood. This is known as "hypoxia." Since acupuncture can encourage circulation and blood flow, it might help prevent such issues from occurring.

In some cases, acupuncture can help delay dialysis by relieving some symptoms. It can even help regulate certain immune disorders and boost immunity by improving the individual's ability to fight off diseases on their own.

No matter what the primary cause of renal failure is, one common cause is renal ischemia and hypoxia which will further harm renal tissues. Acupuncture can promote blood circulation to increase blood and oxygen to the kidneys. By stimulating certain acupoints, additional symptoms like pain, edema, and ecchymosis (when bleeding under the skin causes the skin to bruise) will also be greatly relieved.

Some patients experience dull and persistent pain and have a general feeling of illness due to a buildup of toxins and waste. Acupuncture can stimulate the release of endorphins, the body's natural painkillers. Acupuncture can also soothe the nerves and help block the pain without having to resort to chemicals and other types of painkillers to deal with this persistent pain.

Sometimes, acupuncture can be used along with Micro-Chinese Medicine Osmotherapy for improved treatment. This can lead to anti-inflammation and anti-coagulation (blood clotting) which can help individuals avoid any additional deterioration and protect their remaining kidney function.

CHINESE HERBS FOR KIDNEY DISEASE

There are many different herbs in TCM that are linked to kidney disease and a good trained herbalist will know which ones are meant to be used in the treatment of your disease. Before you start taking any herb or medication, however, it's important to talk to your pharmacist about food/drug interactions that might exist. Your pharmacist is specifically trained to understand these interactions and should be able to answer any questions you may have. The following is a list of these herbs and which ones you might encounter if you visit a herbalist specifically trained in Chinese medicine. Be sure to talk to your healthcare provider before you use herbs as part of your treatment.

You should also only used standardized herbal extracts made by reputable companies and do not use longer than recommended or take more than the recommended dosage. Natural does not mean that it's safe, so use caution. Find out more about specific herbs at the American Botanical Council, www.herbalgram.org or at the National Center for Complementary and Alternative Medicine, at www.nccam.nih.gov

Couch grass

This herb has been used in TCM since around 25 AD. Couch grass is meant to increase urine production and can treat urinary tract infections like urethritis (inflammation of the urethra-the duct in which urine comes out of) and cystitis (also sometimes called a bladder infection). It can also help dissolve kidney stones and relieve pain associated with them. By helping increase urine output, in cases of CKD, it can help remove toxins from your urinary tract and kidneys.

Uva ursi

Uva-ursi is a urinary antiseptic. It has been broadly utilized in herbal medicine since the 2nd century and is primarily used to help disinfect and astringe (clean out) the kidneys, making it particularly useful for those with CKD.

Green tea

Green tea has many different uses. It can reduce bad cholesterol levels and is often used for dieting purposes. It can be used as an astringent (placed on a cotton swab or cotton ball and used directly) or consumed as a drink and is a stimulant. It also has anti-inflammatory properties which makes it useful for individuals with CKD.

Rehmannia

Rehmannia, a root commonly used in TCM, is used to help reduce inflammation within the kidneys. It also detoxifies the liver and can treat hepatitis and rheumatoid arthritis. It's been known to help treat certain autoimmune disorders like lupus as well.

There are also some traditional Chinese herbs that are known for helping control chronic kidney disease and have been used for centuries for the healing of the disease, and not just for the symptoms. Lei Gong Teng, for instance, is an herb that has been used in TCM for many years and some research found that it was effective for helping some forms of polycystic kidney disease, according to a study at Yale University.

Nattokinase, which comes from natto (a fermented soy product) is traditionally used in Japan. It can be found in capsule form and taken twice a day and is sometimes used in TCM for the treatment of CKD in order to help blood circulation. There is a warning, however, that it should be avoided in those who have any kind of blood clotting disorders.

Serrapeptase, which comes from from silkworms, might also help dissolve clots and scar tissues. It can be taken with nattokinase and is another treatment that is often used in TCM.

LIFESTYLE CHANGES

Lifestyle changes can help reduce stress and anxiety, control blood sugar levels, and possibly lower blood pressure which can help take the pressure off the kidneys. Some studies have shown that regular exercise can help improve energy levels for those suffering from kidney disease and strengthen the heart. This is particularly important, given the high death rates that kidney disease patients can have due to heart-related incidences.

Your lifestyle can include exercise, fresh air, and even sunshine. Regular exercise is important and does not have to mean joining a gym or rigorous physical activity. In fact, it can simply mean walking as little as 20 minutes every day. This simple activity can help restore proper circulation. In turn, this can carry oxygen to your cells and transport waste. Exercise will not only improve your circulation, it will also improve your flexibility and energy levels. Many patients with CKD suffer from fatigue and low energy levels and although it sounds like a catch-22, exercise can actually help you have more energy. It just takes getting up and moving around a little bit. If you have mobility issues, then try low-impact exercises such as swimming, walking, and cycling.

When it's possible, it's best to get exercise outside in the fresh air, especially when the sunshine is out. Sunshine, in particular, is important for healing since it contains vitamin D and many individuals with CKD have a vitamin D deficiency. Even spending as little as 15 minutes per day outside without sunscreen can help you increase your vitamin D levels naturally. Getting the benefit of the early morning sunlight can also help reset the body's internal clock and help with insomnia, too.

While you're getting exercise, don't forget to rest as well. Most Americans are actually overworked and don't get as much rest as they should. It's important to get adequate rest and sleep in order for the body to heal. In fact, that's when the body repairs itself-when we are sleeping. Most studies show that we need at least 8 hours of sleep per night. Many people with CKD suffer from insomnia. Some herbs, such as chamomile, valerian, and melatonin, act as natural sedatives and can be taken in tea and capsule form to promote a good night's sleep.

Part of focusing on your lifestyle means that you shouldn't ignore any other underlying health problems you have, even if you are interested in alternative treatment methods of controlling your disease. If you have hypertension, for instance, then it might be necessary to take blood pressure medication regularly until your blood pressure is under control. At that point, then it might be possible to maintain it with natural methods. If you aren't able to completely maintain your blood pressure naturally, then you might at least be able to maintain your stress levels naturally and this can still be helpful in controlling your blood pressure. High blood pressure can cause increased damage to your kidneys, and the medications have a protective effect on your kidneys.

Even with a natural approach, it's important to remember that if you do need to go on dialysis then you should. Although it can be delayed for a time, when it is time to go on dialysis then natural alternative methods can help the body obtain maximum wellness and eliminate certain symptoms so that the individual has the best quality of life.

HERBS & SUPPLEMENTS

When it comes to alternative therapies for kidney disease, herbs and supplements can be important since they are able to help reduce inflammation, flush out toxins, improve overall health, and just generally improve the kidneys' functions. Some common herbs, vitamins, and supplements used to treat kidney disease and its symptoms include: acacia gum, thiamine, omega-3s and fatty acids, grape seed extract, astragalus, milk thistle, carob tree, Vitamin D, Vitamin B6, and ginger. Remember to discuss the use of any herbs or supplements with your provider prior to making any changes.

Acacia gum: Acacia gum might be helpful in treating chronic kidney disease. It contains saccharides and glycoproteins which both have antioxidant properties and can protect the liver and kidneys. Acacia gum might be able to lower blood urea nitrogen. It is also an anti-diarrheal agent, which might be helpful for those individuals who suffer diarrhea as part of their kidney failure.

Pomegranate: Pomegranate is mostly known as a fruit, but can be found in supplement form. Regular use of pomegranate has been shown to reduce inflammation and number of infections in those who are going through dialysis. In 2010, a study carried out by the Technion-Israel Institute of Technology in Haifa, Israel found that the juice alone showed a significantly lower rate of hospitalization caused by infections. The oral presentation, entitled "One Year of Pomegranate Juice Consumption Decreases Oxidative Stress, Inflammation and Incidence of Infections in Hemodialysis Patients" and was presented at the *American Society of Nephrology's 43rd Annual Meeting and Scientific Exposition*, also stated that the 101 dialysis patients who drank the juice experienced reduced inflammation.

Omega-3 fatty acids: Omega 3 fatty acids have a wide variety of health benefits that can't be denied. They've been shown to have healthy effects on both heart rates and blood pressure and now a study has shown their effectiveness in helping certain aspects of kidney disease as well. Many individuals suffering from kidney disease also have hypertension. However, omega-3 fatty acids can lead to improvements in blood pressure, vascular reactivity, and serum lipids. Fish oils in general can suppress inflammations for those with kidney disease and reduce protein loss in urine by as much as 50%.

Vitamin D: According to the 2010 *Mayo Clinic Proceedings* [(85(8): 752–758], most kidney disease patients have inadequate amounts of Vitamin D. However, normal levels of Vitamin D can help reduce some of the symptoms of kidney disease such as depression, insomnia, and muscle weakness and might even prevent the death of kidney cells. Vitamin D supplements, therefore, could be beneficial.

Barberry: Barberry can improve the functioning of the immune system. It is especially good for controlling and preventing kidney stones, as well as for gallbladder issues.

Licorice root: Licorice root is often used in traditional Chinese medicine to enhance other herbs in certain formulas and might be helpful for treating kidney disease, according to the Memorial Sloan-Kettering Cancer Center. The root is used to treat such health issues as constipation, inflammation, and chronic kidney failure. It works as an antioxidant and laxative.

Astragalus: Astragalus might be helpful when it comes to treating advanced kidney disease. It's an herb native to the northern and eastern parts of China and Korea and according to the University of Maryland Medical Center it has been used in traditional Chinese medicine for thousands of years. Its main use has been to reinforce the body against disease. It works by protecting the body against different kinds of stress, including emotional and physical, and repairing damaged tissue. It's an anti-inflammatory, a diuretic, and by lowering the blood pressure can protect the kidneys' function. You can find it in tincture, capsule or tablet form or in a cream that can be applied to the body.

Milk thistle: Milk thistle is a flowering herb and, according to the National Center for Complementary and Alternative Medicine, it's been used for many years to treat lots of different health problems, including high cholesterol levels and kidney failure. As an antioxidant, it might be valuable in helping your kidneys perform better and protecting them from some of the effects of other health issues, such as high blood pressure.

Ginger: Ginger, in its different forms, has been found to be valuable for a lot of different health issues-especially vomiting and nausea. Daily ginger supplements have been known to help with chronic pain, including arthritis. It's also good for the heart and reduces inflammation, but should be avoided if you are taking blood thinners. In April 2004, a study in "Renal Failure" examined whether it could preserve kidney function after ischemia. The study found that dietary supplementation with ginger did provide noteworthy renal protection by activating antioxidants found within the herb.

Grape seed: Grape seed, and grape seed extract, is another multi-purpose herb that has a lot of uses. It might be helpful in treating or preventing kidney failure. Grape seed, also called Vitis vinifera, has been used to treat such problems as edema, nausea, kidney disease, liver disease, and skin infections. Grape seeds contain vitamin E, flavonoids and linoleic acid, all of which have different important healing properties.

Vitamin C: Vitamin C can decrease oxidative stress. Oxidative stress can damage the cellular structure and make the body more inclined to certain diseases. By decreasing your oxidative stress, you might also decrease the amount of damage your kidneys suffer.

Vitamin B6: Vitamin B6 is valuable in helping restore energy levels for those with kidney disease, as well as treating nausea and vomiting. It can also help prevent kidney stones.

Bilberry: In a recent study reported in the *Journal of Agricultural and Food Chemistry* it was found that extracts from bilberry may protect the kidneys from the damaging effects of potassium. The bilberry may also help improve the strength of blood vessels and reduce damage associated with certain diseases, particularly diabetes. The strongest components of the berries are flavonoids, which act as antioxidants. The antioxidants help protect body tissues, especially blood vessels. Rather than allowing dangerous oxidizing agents to bind to body cells, they bind to the antioxidants instead. This way, no serious damage is done to the blood vessels. Bilberries can also help prevent blood clotting and improve circulation.

Chamomile: Chamomile is known for its soothing qualities and many people with chronic diseases take advantage of this benefit. Those with kidney disease are no exception. People with kidney disease especially end-stage kidney disease are more likely to have insomnia. Chamomile tea can be used to soothe the nerves and be used as a mild sedative. Drinking a cup of tea before bedtime can be a good way to encourage sleep and drinking it throughout the day can help anxiety. This can be particularly helpful for those who suffer from insomnia, as many people with chronic kidney disease do. In addition, the amino acid glycine in chamomile tea can be valuable in treating muscle cramps, another common symptom for those with kidney disease or on dialysis. It might also be helpful in lowering high blood pressure.

Echinacea: Echinacea is known for being a natural antibiotic and has been used for naturally healing a variety of infections, from sore throats to minor skin infections. Thanks to these properties, it is also a natural immune system booster as well. As such, it can be helpful to those suffering from kidney disease since it can help strengthen the overall immune system and help protect the body from additional kidney infections.

Glutathione –The positive effects of glutathione are really just now starting to be understood. It is a powerful antioxidant and can be taken directly or your body's stores can be recharged indirectly by getting adequate supplies of Vitamin C. It can help the kidneys detoxify a lot of different chemicals, and might even be valuable in reversing chronic kidney disease, according to a 2004 article in *Nephrology Dialysis Transplantation.*

Hawthorn berry: Hawthorn berries have been known to help boost circulation and improve blood flow to the heart. In Europe, it's highly respected and endorsed by Commission E as an herbal supplement that's valuable in the early stages of heart disease. It has been studied and used for treating such medical conditions as congestive heart failure, valve prolapse, angina, myocarditis, arteriosclerosis and cardiac arrhythmia. Hawthorn berry can also help lower blood pressure. It can be taken as an extract or made into a tea. The powerful antioxidant properties might help lower cholesterol level and reduce the accumulation of fatty plaque in the arteries.

Ginkgo: Gingko bilboa is used to treat many different types of medical conditions but more and more studies are showing its effectiveness when it comes to kidney disease. The extract has most recently been studied in terms of renal disease in a study conducted at a hospital in China. At this clinical trial, it was discovered that individuals with glomerular lesions were improved after taking ginkgo bilboa extract or taking it with other medications. The glomeruli are clusters of blood vessels in which the blood enters the kidneys. The blood is filtered in the glomerulus. Lesions can form on the glomeruli during CKD, however, and this can cause protein and even red blood cells leak into the urine. It might also hinder the elimination of waste and cause edema. Gingko, however, may help eliminate this. If you are taking blood thinners, avoid using gingko.

Lemon balm: Lemon balm (also referred to as Melissa) has been used for insomnia, anxiety, and digestive issues. It could be used for treating certain symptoms caused by kidney disease, especially when combined with other herbs. For instance, lemon balm with valerian can help eliminate insomnia-a common symptom of CKD. It is very gentle and has been known to lower blood pressure, too, when combined with linden flowers which could be valuable for those patients who are suffering from hypertension.

Meadowsweet: Although difficult to locate, meadowsweet is considered one of best herbs for the digestive system. It is a gentle pain reliever without causing the stomach bleeding that certain pain medications like aspirin can cause. It can improve digestion and is often used to treat urinary tract infections, as well as gallstones. It works as a diuretic and has been known to help flush out kidneys and clear up both kidney infections and other urinary tract infections.

Coenzymes: When the kidneys have sustained a lot of damage there is usually a loss of functioning of nephrons to filter the blood. The nephrons are basically the fundamental structural units of the kidneys. They perform important jobs such as sustaining the concentrations of water and soluble substances in the blood as well as controlling blood volume and blood pressure. When nephrons are damaged, the remaining nephrons must work even harder. When the kidneys are overworked, it's called a state of hyperfiltration. They're most likely to fail at this point. The coenzyme Q10 and L-carnitine can provide energy on the cellular level to the nephrons. This will offer support to the healthy nephrons and help them keep up with the body's demands.

PROBIOTICS

Waste products can become toxic if they accumulate in the blood and aren't removed. This can be harmful to many of the body's organs, especially the kidneys. When the kidneys become impaired, the waste can buildup in the bloodstream and this is dangerous to the body. Probiotics are dietary supplements that help break down the wastes that have diffused from the bloodstream into the digestive system. The wastes are then used as nutrients. Probiotics can be live organisms like bacteria or yeast and many people believe that they create a healthy atmosphere within the digestive system since they help the body digest some foods. More and more people are finding the benefits to probiotics as they help regulate the digestive system and create a healthier gut.

Studies show that a lot of digestive disorders occur when the sense of balance between the "good" bacteria and the "bad" bacteria within the intestines becomes disturbed. This is something that usually happens after an infection or when a person takes antibiotics, which can kill not only the bad bacteria but the good bacteria as well, and allow yeast to overgrow. Taking probiotics can help restore that balance. Some studies show that probiotics might be able to help people maintain a stronger digestive system as well as a stronger immune system. In fact, in cultures where the hygiene is very good, there has actually been an increase in allergic diseases and autoimmune diseases which could be an unintentional offshoot of killing the good bacteria within the digestive system.

Some probiotics can make use of uric acid, creatinine, and other toxins as its nutrients for growing purposes. As they're expanding, they can create a greater dispersion of these toxins from the circulating blood across the intestinal walls into the bowel. This can then be excreted along with the rest of the waste.

A regular healthy digestive tract has around 400 kinds of probiotic bacteria that control the growth of dangerous bacteria and promote a healthy digestive system. Good bacteria are important not just for bowel health, but for overall health. The good intestinal bacteria can profit health by synthesizing vitamins and fighting against infections. Good bacteria might also help prevent certain types of bowel cancer, bowel disease, and peptic ulcers.

ADDITIONAL THERAPIES

In many alternative therapies, a holistic approach is taken. This means that not only is the body treated, but the mind and spirit are as well. Alternative therapies can include regular colonic irrigations, magnesium salts and castor oil packs over the kidneys, color therapy, reflexology, meditation, aromatherapy, massage, and craniosacral treatments. Some of these can be used in conjunction with one another in order to offer the most benefits.

In a holistic approach, treatment will combine the body, mind, and spirit. Hippocrates is considered the father of medicine and in the 4th century BC he wrote of healing the entire patient and not just the disease. A lot of alternative treatments rely on this method today. As a result, some alternative treatments are preventative and nourishing and meant to keep the body and mind in balance so that diseases do not get worse, or don't happen in the first place. Sometimes, alternative treatments are carried out with the belief that the body is actually capable of healing itself if given the proper aids and atmosphere.

MEDITATION

Meditation is an excellent way to relax both your body and mind. It's also a good way to eliminate any tension that might exist within you. Studies show that stress can wreck havoc on your health and actually cause health problems, especially within your digestive system, but can even lower your immune system. By lowering your stress levels you might be able to boost your immune system, regulate your digestive system, and improve your overall health.

At the 2013 American Society of Nephrology's Kidney Week 2013 meeting, research was presented by Emory University School of Medicine that showed that meditation may decrease blood pressure in individuals with CKD. By using only 14 minutes of mindfulness meditation per day, blood pressure was lowered in patients with CKD Stage 3 and hypertension.

Mindfulness meditation encourages the practitioner to be "mindful" and basically focuses on being in the present and being aware of your thoughts and actions and what's going on around you. Rather than trying to get the individual to change, it encourages them to be in the moment and experience the life that is happening within them and around them, instead of being concerned with what might happen in the future or upset about things that occurred in the past.

Practicing meditation:

First, it's important to find a peaceful spot to relax it. It might be your bedroom, your office, or a corner of your living room. It should be quiet and hopefully free of distractions.

Next, get comfortable. Some people find it easier to sit on a cushion. You want something that won't move around too much. Your posture should be straight without being stiff. Try not to get into anything uncomfortable since you'll be prone to focus on that, and not the breathing and visualization, both of which are important in meditation. If you're sitting on the floor or a cushion, cross your legs in front of you.

Rest your hands on your thighs and lightly close your eyes. They shouldn't be completely closed. You don't want to stare or focus your gaze on anything in particular; you simply want to let your eyes "rest." The idea is to let the front of your body be "open."

For a few minutes, you want to simply sit still and experience the environment around you. The idea is to let your mind become "aware" of its surroundings. Next, you will work on your breathing.

Focus on taking a breath in and a breath out. Don't manipulate your breathing; just pay attention to the way you breathe. Pay careful attention to your chest rising and falling and the air moving in and out of you. Do this for several minutes-breathe and notice your breathing without trying to control it.

Lastly, consider your thoughts. As your thoughts begin focusing and sometimes try to run amok, gently try to swat them away and turn your attention back to your breathing. Don't judge your thoughts or worry about them, just acknowledge them and then use your breathing to anchor you back. The more you practice this, the easier it will become.

You can practice mindful meditation for about 15 to 20 minutes every day to get the most benefits. In the beginning, it might be difficult, but the more you practice it, the easier you'll find it becomes. Another benefit of learning to meditate is that you will find it much easier to focus on activities in general and not let y our mind wander so much when you are focused.

NATUROPATHY TREATMENTS

In naturopathy, there are some common treatments that are used as far as kidney disease is concerned. These include the use of kidney packs and fomentation (as described below). In some naturopathic treatments, there is a fruit fast for 5-7 days. During that time, warm-water enemas and herbal enemas with herbs beneficial to the kidneys are administered on a daily basis, along with hip-baths. This should be done with caution under the instruction of a knowledgeable medical professional.

ADDITIONAL FORMS OF NATUROPATHIC TREATMENTS INCLUDE:
Kidney pack: A kidney pack is a combination of a hot and cold pack. Using a cotton cloth, you cover a hot water bottle and place it over your middle to lower back. At the same time, an ice bag is placed over your lower part of the chest bone and stomach and a dry cotton cloth is placed over this. Both of these are left on for about an hour every day.

Fomentation : Fomentation increases blood circulation to the abdominal organs, boosts metabolic functions, reduces inflammation, and soothes the nervous system. It also eases anxiety and relieves pain and indigestion and calms the urinary organs. A fomentation bag (a hot water bottle) is filled with hot water and placed on the abdomen covering the last rib, extending up to the line of the liver and spleen. At the same time, a cold bag is placed on the lumbar spine. The bags are left on for about an hour every day.

A hot castor oil pack might be effective at relaxing cramping or painful muscles which might be helpful for those who experience pain with their kidney disease and are looking for alternative methods of pain relief. The muscles absorb the oil through the lymphatic circulation. This helps stimulate the immune function. Castor oil packs have also been known to help constipation, inflammation, inflamed joints, and kidney stones, too. You can find out more about castor oil packs by going to this video that explains how to do them.

http://www.renaldiethq.com/go/castoroilpack

MASSAGE

Massage is an excellent way to relax, but it can also be a good treatment option as well. In fact, it is actually one of the oldest treatment options in the world. Massage has good therapeutic effects on both chronic and functional diseases. It can relieve symptoms, make patients feel more comfortable, and improve their quality of life. Of course, it's important to ensure that you're getting a massage by a licensed professional. To get the best and most lasting effects, have regular massages.

Massage for chronic kidney disease can help encourage blood circulation and increase blood flow within the kidneys to help improve kidney functions. Some patients find that after getting regular massages they have improved digestion and chronic pain relief, something that many people suffer with chronic kidney disease. An improvement in these symptoms helps improve their overall quality of life.

Most people do not suffer any side effects from massage, which makes it a suitable alternative treatment for the majority of patients. In fact, since it's a relaxing treatment and has the side effect of a release of tension it's actually a treatment that most everyone can enjoy.

Full body massages are the most common types of massages that are sought, but hand massages are also beneficial to those suffering from CKD. The hands have trigger points on them and these can correspond to organs (using reflexology). By pressing on these trigger points, it's possible to strengthen that organ and affect the system it's linked to.

Hand massage might be able to stimulate the kidneys and revitalize renal tissues to promote the generation of new tissues. This can boost blood circulation and increase blood flow to alleviate renal ischemia and hypoxia. It might also offer the kidneys more vital nutrients and even improve filtering so that the kidneys are able to eliminate toxic wastes. In addition, hand massage can affect high blood pressure, headaches, and insomnia, all common symptoms of CKD. Remember, this is mainly for symptomatic relief, not a cure.

REFLEXOLOGY

Like massage, reflexology relies on pressure points on the body. However, there is an art to reflexology that goes a step further than traditional massage. Reflexology believes that certain trigger points actually causes the immune system and nervous system to act in a certain manner. The main foot reflexes for the kidneys are close to the middle of the soles of the feet, although there are there are several acupoints on the feet and almost all internal organs and every system in the entire body have analogous reflex zones in the feet.

Several major studies around the world have found benefits regarding reflexology and patients suffering from kidney disease. For instance, it has been discovered that reflexology has an increase in blood flow to both intestines and the kidneys. It has also demonstrated positive changes to kidney functions to those on dialysis. Anxiety and blood pressure have been decreased in those suffering from kidney disease and according to the book *Evidence-Based Reflexology for Health Professionals and Researchers: The Reflexology Research Series* by Barbara and Kevin Kunz (2008), 27 different studies have shown a marked decrease in pain for those suffering from chronic kidney disease by getting reflexology.

Reflexology has been successfully used amongst chronic disease patients. It can be used to help relieve some symptoms and prevent other symptoms from occurring. For those that have advanced kidney disease, it can also be an important harmonizing therapy.

Reflexology is a treatment that should be performed by a licensed therapist who has specialized training and certification. The therapist is trained to massage the trigger points on the feet that correspond with the kidneys. During the treatment, blood circulation is encouraged by massaging the acupoints. Since renal failure can occur when blood flow to the kidneys is interrupted, blood circulation is important. By putting pressure on the right areas, blood flow to the kidneys can be encouraged, which is beneficial to those with CKD.

Most individuals have reflexology about 2-4 times per week for kidney disease. For those with acute renal failure, appointments might be more regular. The pace of the massage might be very quick for those whose disease is severe while the pace might be slower for those facing a chronic disease. After the massage, it is usually suggested that the patient drink at least a full glass of water to help eliminate any toxins.

YOGA

Yoga is another relaxing exercise that might be helpful in treating kidney disease, both for its stress relieving techniques and for its elements of physical activity. Yoga provides gentle stretching and twisting to the spine and body which naturally massages the kidneys and can smooth the muscles around them. In addition, during yoga individuals practice meditation which can also help release tension and stress.

Certain yoga positions are known to help kidney functions. They include:

Bhujangasana (also known as the "Cobra" pose): Lie on your stomach with your arms on either side of you. All your weight should be on your hands, thighs, and legs. Slowly, raise your head and your chest from the ground up to your navel. Much like a push up with the upper half or your body raised and your hips/legs remaining on the ground.

This pose helps treat uterine disorders as well as liver disorders, the gallbladder, and slipped discs.

Ardha matsendrasana (also known as the "Half Spinal Twist" or the "Half Lord of the Fishes" pose):

Sit on a yoga mat with your spine straight and feet together and your legs outstretched. Raise your right leg and place it against the outside of your left knee with your soles firmly on the floor. Stretch your left arm out and place your fingers on the toes of your right foot. Place your right arm around the back of your waist so that your palm rests on your left hip bone. Your spine should be straight. Look over your right shoulder. Don't slouch. Remain in this position for as long as you can, and then gradually relax.

This pose stimulates the liver, heart, lungs, kidneys and spleen.

Crescent lunge:

Stand straight. Place your right leg in front of you in a 90 degree angle. Stretch your left leg out behind in you in a straight line. This will make a "high lunge." Your stomach should be lifted in and up while your chest is lifted. Reach your arms straight up over your head. Place your palms together. Hold for a count of 5-10 at first, increasing to 30 over time.

AROMATHERAPY

Aromatherapy, the art of using essential oils for their healing aromas in the treatment of various diseases, can also be used an as alternative treatment for kidney disease. It's important to use caution with aromatherapy. Undiluted essential oils shouldn't be applied directly to your skin since they're too concentrated and this could cause a chemical burn. Also, not all oils are meant to be used for CKD and some scents can cause adverse reactions. Some oils you should avoid include: black pepper, juniper, licorice, fennel, and sandalwood. Since essential oils are absorbed through the skin, using too much of an oil can result in an overdose. When in doubt, go to an expert. Most massage therapists are skilled in the art of using essential oils and can act as aromatherapists. You can always ask the massage therapist upfront or look for one who can also act in this capacity.

Juniper Oil

Juniper oil is one of the most popular oils to use during the treatment of CKD. It is steam distilled from the aerial parts of the juniper shrub, as well as the stems, leaves, and flowers. Juniper oil to similar to fennel oil and is a diuretic. It's helpful because it encourages urination which helps flush out harmful toxins from the kidneys. As a result, it's valuable for patients with kidney disease who might be suffering from edema due to chronic renal failure. It can also help reducing blood pressure and eliminate extra sodium and toxins such as uric acid.

Juniper oil should be used as a homeopathic dose. Since the kidneys are in such a weakened state from chronic kidney disease, some of the most powerful oils may be too much for them to cope with. Juniper is so effective at removing unwanted "garbage" from your body that it would only put more pressure on the kidneys. In this case, we use what is called a homeopathic dose. That is 1/15th of a drop. It sounds complicated to create but it is not. Take a carrier oil (such as sunflower oil), and count out 14 drops. Add to it on drop of essential oil. Then use one drop of the mix – there you have it!

Juniper oil might also remove blood toxins and act as a blood purifier. It can remove heavy metals, pollutants, and compounds and hormones produced by the body as well as foreign toxins that accidentally get into the blood. In the process, it supports the kidneys by allowing them to function the way they're supposed to.

German chamomile is another essential oil that is used in aromatherapy for CKD. It contains a lot of antioxidants and helps eliminate free radicals from the body and fights inflammation. In one study, chamomile oil was able to stop the growth of certain cancer cells while not causing any harm to the healthy cells around it. Chamomile oil is often diluted with olive oil or grape seed oil and massaged over the kidneys for 5-10 minutes, at least once a day for detoxification.

Finally, lavender oil is the most efficacious oil in the kit. It is very soothing and relaxing, as well as relieving pain. Lavender is especially helpful to calm difficult days and relax. In moments of anxiety, using lavender can help to relax the patient. It also helps greatly with insomnia, something many with chronic kidney disease suffer from.

When using aromatherapy, more is not better. Use a mixture of just 1-2 drops and combine with a carrier oil (such as an unscented lotion or sunflower oil). Rub it into the skin and you will see that it makes it's way to the area where it's needed. You don't have to smell it strongly to have it work, either. Be especially cautious and start slowly but expand to see if you can help your symptoms.

CRANIOSACRAL TREATMENTS

Craniosacral therapy (CST), also known as craniosacral treatments, supports the nervous system by balancing the cerebrospinal fluid that surrounds and protects the brain and spinal cord. The fluid moves all the way from the skull to the tailbone and by adding balancing to it, the nervous system is able to find harmony and settle down. This allows the body to function properly since the nervous system is responsible for so much of how the body works. CST has been used to treat many different types of conditions, from brain dysfunctions to migraines, chronic headaches, dyslexia, and chronic pain. It's also been used to treat other nervous system disorders. It can be helpful in treating CKD due to the fact that practitioners believe that all the bodily systems work off one another and that the digestive system is closely interwoven with the nervous system and that if one gets out of balance, the other will as well.

To receive treatment, patients lay on a table and the medical practitioner gently touches their body and feels for the pulse of their cerebrospinal fluid. In order to help balance out the fluid's rhythm they will apply tender pressure to certain parts of the patient's head, spine, and tailbone. The treatment will not hurt or be uncomfortable to the patient. Although the treatment itself will be mostly physical, part of it will be based on intuition. As the practitioner feels for the fluid's pulse, they will "listen" to the patient's body as well. Much of the CST relies on the patient releasing old emotions that the nervous system might be holding onto that is causing the body both physical and mental pain. The practitioner can help the body release these pains and emotions.

A typical session will run about half an hour. Most patients end up feeling relaxed afterwards. Some even end up falling asleep. For those who suffer from CKD, treatments might help reduce edema and chronic pain-symptoms that are associated with chronic kidney disease. Although most patients seek treatment from a practitioner, a family member or loved one can learn to perform the treatments at home for the individual.

AYURVEDA

Ayurveda is a holistic approach to health and one of the oldest healing sciences in the world. It developed in India thousands of years ago and many of its principles are still applied today all over the world. Some patients with chronic kidney disease turn to this approach since it treats the whole patient and not just the disease itself. When it comes to kidney failure, most of kidney's function has been lost. As a result, a lot of wastes and toxins can build up within the body. Plus, electrolyte imbalance, immune disorders and additional complications can occur as well. In Ayurveda, balance within the body, mind, and consciousness is maintained through lifestyle and diet and this can, in turn, treat the kidney failure and restore some kidney function. Many patients find that by using the Ayurvedic approach they are able to enjoy more energy and a stronger immune system, too.

Ayurveda can help slightly-damaged kidneys repair themselves and achieve improved functioning. It might also help normalize creatinine levels to near their regular levels. Damaged nephrons can also be permanently controlled with the help of Ayurveda treatments, in some cases. Ayurvedic treatment can also help the patient maintain their levels of sodium and potassium since even small imbalances could cause harm to the patient.

When it comes to Ayurvedic treatment for kidney failure, it is carried out through the use of herbs and what is referred to as "medications."

These different herbs have various properties in the treatment of chronic kidney disease which include, but are not limited to:

- Acting as diuretics
- Anti-inflammatory
- Regulating blood pressure
- Pain reducing
- Improving skin problems
- Antibiotics
- Reducing cholesterol levels
- Boosting immune system

In treating kidney failure, it is first determined whether or not there is an underlying cause, such as diabetes or hypertension. If the patient smokes, then they'll be recommended to stop. Treatment will commence on that underlying condition with the expectation that the kidney's function will resume to a healthier level once the underlying condition has been cleared up.

Herbal medicines will then be administered to treat the symptoms and any damage that has already been done to the damaged kidneys. Ayurveda does use such practices as hip baths, kidney packs, and fomentations to help alleviate symptoms and reduce inflammation on the kidneys as well. If the damage, however, is too severe then dialysis might be suggested in the event that Ayurveda practices are not enough.

COLOR THERAPY

Color therapy is an alternative therapy that is gaining in popularity in many different kinds of holistic healing center. Also referred to as "osmotherapy," it relies on the idea that colors can influence certain areas of our lives, including energy levels, mood, health, emotion, and our mental states. Colors are meant to be associated with different chakras, or seven energy centers, according to Ayurveda, although color therapy has also evolved outside of Ayurveda and has been expanded upon using many of the older principles. Practitioners do not have to be licensed in the United States, although there are certification courses available.

Some individuals use color therapy to help with their kidney disease since they believe that their chakras are out of balance and the different colors can help eliminate pain, boost circulation, eliminate toxins from the kidneys, and lower blood pressure.

The different colors have different corresponding meanings. For "weak" kidneys (kidneys that have lost function) violet light is best. Shining violet light on them, 30 to 60 minutes at a time, at least twice a day, is ideal.

Other colors associated with color therapy include:

- **Red**
Red is associated with the spine, hips and legs. It is a warm color and is stimulating. It stimulates physical energy and boosts circulation.

- **Orange**
Orange is associated with happiness and optimism and is considered good for depression. It is linked to the sacral chakra and is thought to benefit the kidneys, urinary tract and the reproductive organs. It can help stimulate digestion and relieve gas and digestion and is beneficial for chronic kidney disease since it stimulates the kidneys' function. Too much of it might cause exhaustion, however, so it should be limited for those with CKD who have low energy levels.

- **Yellow**
Yellow is linked to the solar plexus chakra. A bright color, it's also the brightest color and is considered a happy one. It's very strong. An imbalance in this chakra could encourage confusion or fear. The solar plexus chakra is also thought to influence the digestive system. It helps stimulate digestion and gastric juices so it should be used for any digestive uses other than the spleen.

- **Blue**

Blue is a soothing color and can help insomnia, anxiety, throat problems, high blood pressure, and migraines. It can also be used for pain relief.

Color therapy can be used in different ways, not just by using lights. It can also be used by visualizing different colors while meditating and drinking different colored water. The lights can be colored by using colored bulbs or by filtering the sunlight through glass or cellophane. Some people treat their kidneys by shining the lights at close range on their skin for short periods of time several times a day. However, it's important to careful when doing this, especially when using warm lights since this could cause burns, depending on the type of bulb.

TAKING PRECAUTIONS

It's important to remember to follow any instructions that your doctor has given you. In addition, keep in mind that some herbs can be dangerous to consume in general, while others are specifically not safe for those with kidney disease. Herbs that are generally considered unsafe for those with chronic kidney disease include: blue cohosh, aloe, noni juice, horse chestnut, sassafras, and wormwood plant, juniper berry (the herb, not the oil), lovage root, and white sandalwood. Of course, before embarking on any dietary changes or exercise regimens, it's important to talk to your doctor or dietitian, especially if you have any other underlying health concerns such as diabetes or high blood pressure.

There are some herbs that might make good diuretics, which is helpful, but could also cause kidney irritation or even damage to your kidneys. These include juniper berries and bucha leaves. Juniper berries are safe as long as they are used as an oil in aromatherapy but they shouldn't be used in tea form or consumed. Parsley capsules are another herb that can cause kidney irritation when consumed since they can have dangerous side effects to those who suffer from kidney failure. Parsley used in cooking is fine.

Sometimes, certain herbs can cause interactions with different medications. Even though the herbs themselves aren't dangerous, when they are mixed with certain chemicals the contraindications are harmful. St. Johns Wort is one such herb that can have side effects when mixed when many kidney medications, as are Echinacea, ginkgo, and blue cohosh. If you've had a transplant or are taking any medications then always check to make sure that you're not at risk of having any contraindications at developing complications between the herbs and any medications you're on. You can talk to your doctor or pharmacist about this. Remember to discuss all the herbs and over the counter medications you take with your doctor.

Even though herbs are natural, they can still be powerful. Valerian and chamomile are natural sedatives and can make you very sleepy. If you're taking them or lemon balm (Melissa) or even using them in the essential oil form then you might want to have someone else around to do the driving or be alert for you. They might also heighten the effect of any other medications you're taking that have a sedative effect so keep that in mind as well.

When you're looking for an acupuncturist, reflexologist, and massage therapist remember that they must be certified and that there are certain standards they have to adhere to. Acupuncturists are certified by the National Certification Commission of Acupuncture and Oriental Medicine. You can search for certified professionals in your area on their website at http://www.nccaom.org/. Likewise, reflexologists are certified by the American Reflexology Certification Board (ARCB), although they can receive training and degrees from different schools and programs from across the country. Massage therapists must be certified by the National Certification Board for Therapeutic Massage and Bodywork. To maintain their certification, massage therapists must attend regular training sessions and keep up-to-date on their license. You can find more information, and look for therapists, at http://www.ncbtmb.org/.

Despite the fact that naturopathic medicine sounds alternative to many, it actually is regulated and the professionals who practice it are licensed. There are currently 17 states, the District of Columbia, as well as Puerto Rico and the US Virgin Islands that have regulation laws for naturopathic doctors. Naturopathic doctors must graduate from an accredited 4-year residential naturopathic medical school. They must also pass an all-embracing postdoctoral board examination (NPLEX) to receive a license. They also have to fulfill certain state-mandated continuing education requirements every year, and these can differ depending on the state they practice in. You can find a naturopath near you at: http://www.naturopathic.org/.

When in doubt, it's always better to seek a professional, even when you're seeking alternative forms of treatment for your kidney disease.

Even better if you can find someone with skill and experience helping those with kidney failure. Be sure to ask if they have some experience with people with chronic illnesses.

CONCLUSION

Many patients enjoy having a safe and natural holistic treatment for chronic kidney disease. Alternative treatments often take a natural approach to overall health and look at the patient as a whole, treating not only the symptoms but underlying health concerns that can leave the individual feeling full of energy and overall wellbeing. Many of the alternative CKD treatments treat symptoms associated with the disease.

For patients who are in the early stage of kidney disease, their bodies might be brought back into balance so that the progression of the disease might be slowed down. For patients who are in the later stages of the disease and have very compromised kidneys, alternative treatments might keep their kidneys functioning with a simpler and natural maintenance course of therapy. A holistic approach and natural medicine can often control blood pressure, inflammation and cholesterol levels and improve kidney function without the oftentimes dangerous side effects that prescription drugs can have.

When you're looking at alternative treatments for kidney disease, keep in mind that not all treatments are suited for all stages of the disease. Some treatments are not suitable for end-stage renal disease, especially if you're taking certain medications that might dangerously interact with certain herbs and supplements. Still, many of the alternative treatments can offer vast amounts of relief and support to those with CKD and many patients find that the unconventional approaches often suit them well.

If you find this book helpful but want more specifics about aromatherapy, reflexology, and craniosacral therapy, you might be interested in our study guide:

Caring for Renal Patients: http://www.amazon.com/Headquarters-Disease-Patients-Educational-Worksheets/dp/B00LZ2ICPW/

OTHER TITLES BY MATHEA FORD:

Mathea Ford, Author Page (all books):

http://www.amazon.com/Mathea-Ford/e/B008E1E7IS/

The Kidney Friendly Diet Cookbook

http://www.amazon.com/Kidney-Friendly-Diet-Cookbook-PreDialysis-ebook/dp/B00BC7BGPI/

Create Your Own Kidney Diet Plan

http://www.amazon.com/Create-Your-Kidney-Diet-Plan-ebook/dp/B009PSN3R0/

Living with Chronic Kidney Disease - Pre-Dialysis

http://www.amazon.com/Living-Chronic-Kidney-Disease-Pre-Dialysis-ebook/dp/B008D8RSAQ/

Eating a Pre-Dialysis Kidney Diet - Calories, Carbohydrates, Fat & Protein, Secrets To Avoid Dialysis

http://www.amazon.com/Eating-Pre-Dialysis-Kidney-Diet-Carbohydrates-ebook/dp/B00DU2JCHM/

Eating a Pre-Dialysis Kidney Diet - Sodium, Potassium, Phosphorus and Fluids, A Kidney Disease Solution

http://www.amazon.com/Eating-Pre-Dialysis-Kidney-Diet-Phosphorus-ebook/dp/B00E2U8VMS/

Eating Out On a Kidney Diet: Pre-dialysis and Diabetes: Ways To Enjoy Your Favorite Foods

http://www.amazon.com/Eating-Out-Kidney-Diet-Pre-dialysis/dp/0615928781/

Kidney Disease: Common Labs and Medical Terminology: The Patient's Perspective

http://www.amazon.com/Kidney-Disease-Terminology-Perspective-Pre-Dialysis/dp/0615931804/

Dialysis: Treatment Options for the Progression to End Stage Renal Disease

http://www.amazon.com/Dialysis-Treatment-Options-Progression-Disease/dp/0615932258/

Mindful Eating For A Pre-Dialysis Kidney Diet: Healthy Attitudes Toward Food and Life

http://www.amazon.com/Mindful-Eating-Pre-Dialysis-Kidney-Diet/dp/0615933475/

The Emotional Challenges Of Coping with Chronic Kidney Disease

http://www.amazon.com/Emotional-Challenges-Chronic-Disease-Dialysis-ebook/dp/B00H6SYQG8/

Heart Healthy Living with Kidney Disease: Lowering Blood Pressure

http://www.amazon.com/Heart-Healthy-Living-Kidney-Disease/dp/0615936059/

Exercising with Chronic Kidney Disease: Solutions To An Active Lifestyle

http://www.amazon.com/Exercising-Chronic-Kidney-Disease-Solutions/dp/0615936342/

Sexuality and Chronic Kidney Disease For Men and Women: A Path To Better Understanding

http://www.amazon.com/Sexuality-Chronic-Kidney-Disease-Women/dp/0615960197/

Anemia and Chronic Kidney Disease: Signs, Symptoms, and Treatment for Anemia in Kidney Failure

http://www.amazon.com/Anemia-Chronic-Kidney-Disease-Treatment/dp/0692201416/

Positive Beginnings: The Dialysis Breakfast Cookbook

http://www.amazon.com/Positive-Beginnings-Dialysis-Breakfast-Cookbook/dp/069227958X/

Sign up for our email list to learn of new titles right away!

http://www.renaldiethq.com/go/email/

Made in the USA
Middletown, DE
21 June 2017